The Flavorful Fix:
A Savvy Guide to Supercharge Your Health with Nutrient-Dense Whole Foods

Savor the Goodness and Reap the Benefits of a Deliciously Nutritious Diet

MARLEEN D. ANDERSON

Content

Chapter four

Chapter five

Chapter six

Conclusion

Appendix

MARLEEN D. ANDERSON

The Flavorful Fix: A Savvy Guide to Supercharge Your Health with Nutrient-Dense Whole Food

Introduction

Nutrient-dense eating has become increasingly popular in recent years, and for a good reason. Consuming whole-foods rich in nutrients is essential for optimal health and wellness. Nutrient density is a term used to describe the amount of nutrition in a specific volume of food.

Foods considered nutrient-dense contain a high level of essential vitamins, minerals, and other nutrients while having a lower caloric value. These often include super foods that are known for their health benefits. Energy-dense foods have a higher caloric value but contain fewer nutrients relative to their volume.

Nutrient-dense foods are rich in essential vitamins, minerals, and phytochemicals that are vital for sustaining excellent health. This book aims to help you understand how nutrient-dense foods provide your body with the essential building blocks needed for optimal health. We explore how whole-foods are rich in the nutrients your body needs and how their consumption can improve your overall health.

While we live and preform in your daily life, it is important to note that the influence of processing on nutrient density cannot be ignored. Processing foods can lead to the loss of essential nutrient. When you consume whole-foods, you're consuming foods in their natural state, which means they retain their essential nutrients. The book delves deeper into the impact of processing on nutrient density and why eating whole-foods is vital for good health.

Are you looking for practical ideas for developing a nutrient-dense diet? Our book offers meal planning and preparation instructions to help you achieve this goal. We discuss the numerous types of whole-foods and their specific nutritional benefits, such as fruits, vegetables, whole grains, legumes, nuts, and seeds. We also present advice for how to incorporate them into your diet. We'll also cover how to make whole-foods a sustainable part of your lifestyle so that you can enjoy the advantages for the long term.

Did you know that there is a link between whole-foods and disease prevention, longevity, the environment, and social justice? The newest scientific findings suggest that consuming whole-foods can reduce the risk of chronic diseases such as heart disease, diabetes, and cancer. We'll also explore how whole-foods might increase cognitive function, physical performance, and longevity.

Finally, we understand that sometimes it's challenging to know where to start when it comes to eating whole-foods. That's why this book includes delicious whole-foods recipes and meal plans to help you get started on your path to optimal health. We've included a wide variety of recipes for breakfast, lunch, dinner, snacks, and desserts that are easy to create and delightful to consume.

Whether you're wanting to reduce weight, boost energy, or just feel better in your own skin, this book is a comprehensive guide that will provide you with practical ideas, advice, and delicious recipes to make your journey to optimal health a success. With the correct information and the appropriate mindset, you'll be on your way to optimal health in no time.

CHAPTER ONE

Understanding the Science of Nutrient Density

This chapter provides an in-depth understanding of how whole-foods are packed with essential vitamins, minerals, and phytochemicals, and how these micronutrients and phytochemicals play a vital role in maintaining good health. It also covers the impact of processing on nutrient density, and the importance of consuming unprocessed whole-foods to ensure that you're getting the most nutritious bang for your buck. This chapter sets the stage for the rest of the book by providing a solid understanding of the scientific basis of whole-foods nutrition and lays the foundation for the practical strategies discussed in later chapters.

THE MECHANISM OF NUTRIENT DENSITY

You're hungry, and dinner is still a few hours away, you're contemplating a snack. You have two options to choose from, an apple or a cupcake, which are approximately the same size and can serve as a quick snack before you return to your work. Which one do you choose?

Hopefully, you choose the apple instead of the cupcake. The apple contains numerous vitamins, fiber, and phytochemicals and provides approximately 80 calories. To keep you feeling full until dinner, the fiber content in apples can be helpful. The cupcake has calories—lots of calories. In fact, the cupcake has more than 300 calories, but it doesn't have many nutrients.

Consuming a sugary donut only provides about one gram of fiber, which doesn't have the ability to make you feel satiated for long. As a result, you may feel inclined to consume a second or third donut. Although it may taste delicious at the moment, your body could potentially suffer from the after-effects of this instantaneous indulgence.

WHAT FOODS ARE NUTRIENT-DENSE?

Foods with a high nutritional value include those packed with the following nutrients: calcium, potassium, fiber, magnesium, and any vitamins. When we try adding in more natural, plant-based foods, such as non-starchy vegetables (leafy greens, carrots, tomatoes, and broccoli), a colorful variety of fruits (bananas, berries, pineapple, grapes and melons), whole grains (oats, quinoa, and brown/wild rice), along with all beans, legumes, nuts and seeds.

Fish and low-fat meats are also rich in protein and iron, and are a great way to improve your diet. Though, too much red meat and pork may have a serious impact, as these can be high in cholesterol, though a diet that contains a controlled amount of meat and fish also has notable benefits.

While dairy products can provide essential nutrients like calcium, vitamins, and fiber, they should still be consumed in moderation due to their potential to be high in fats. Opt for skim, low-fat or fat-free variations. Individuals with a dairy allergy (or those that simply want to limit their dairy intake) may want to explore dairy-free options. Alternative milk and dairy products made from nuts, soy, and oats are becoming increasingly popular.

WHAT ARE THE BENEFITS OF EATING NUTRIENT-DENSE FOODS?

Eating a wholesome diet rich in nutrients is crucial for your overall health, particularly as you get older. By consuming more nutrients, you'll be taking in more purposeful calories, which can assist in maintaining a healthy weight and promoting mental and gut health.

To combat low energy levels caused by anemia, iron-rich foods such as spinach and eggs can be beneficial. Magnesium aids in regulating sleep, as well as promoting healthy blood pressure, bones, and heart.

As we age, proteins such as fish and chicken are essential for building and preserving muscle mass.. In order to maintain strong bones and muscles, calcium is important and it can be found primarily in dairy products. Additionally, fish is rich in omega-3 fatty acids, which can aid in preventing heart attacks and maintaining cognitive and joint health.

However, it is crucial to note that guided eating is key. Treating oneself to dessert or favorite cuisine every once in a while can make life more enjoyable

THE IMPORTANCE OF NUTRIENT DENSITY IN OPTIMAL HEALTH

Nutrient density refers to the amount of essential vitamins, minerals, and phytochemicals that a food contains in relation to its calorie content. Whole-foods, such as fruits, vegetables, whole grains, legumes, and nuts, are typically high in nutrient density and are considered to be the most nutritious foods available.

The human body requires a wide variety of micronutrients and phytochemicals to function properly. These micronutrients and phytochemicals, such as vitamins, minerals, antioxidants and phytochemicals, play a critical role in maintaining good health and preventing chronic diseases. They help to maintain a healthy immune system, support proper growth and development, protect against oxidative stress and inflammation, and promote overall well-being.

When a diet is low in nutrient density, it is often high in calories and low in essential nutrients. This type of diet can lead to nutrient deficiencies and an increased risk of chronic diseases such as obesity, heart disease, diabetes, and cancer. On the other hand, a diet rich in nutrient-dense whole-foods can help to meet the body's nutritional needs and promote optimal health.

Nutrient density is essential for optimal health and consuming whole-foods is the best way to ensure that your diet is rich in essential nutrients. Whole-foods are packed with essential vitamins, minerals, and phytochemicals that are vital for maintaining good health and preventing chronic diseases.

Eating a diet that is high in nutrient density can help to reduce the risk of chronic diseases, promote healthy growth and development, support a healthy immune system and provide energy to fuel our daily activities. Furthermore, nutrient-dense whole-foods are often low in calories, which can help with weight management.

Nutrient-dense whole-foods can also help to improve our overall well-being. Whole-foods are often high in fiber which can help to keep us full and satisfied, and they also provide us with a sense of pleasure when we eat them.

Whole-foods are not only good for our body but also for our mind and soul.

Eating a diet high in nutrient-dense whole-foods is essential for optimal health, and it should be the foundation of our diet. By including a variety of nutrient-dense whole-foods in our diet, we can ensure that we are getting the essential nutrients our body needs for optimal health and well-being.

WHAT ARE MICRONUTRIENTS AND PHYTOCHEMICALS?

Micronutrients are essential vitamins and minerals that our body needs in small amounts to function properly, such as vitamins A, C, D, E, K, and B vitamins and minerals like iron, zinc, iodine, and selenium. Phytochemicals are naturally occurring compounds in plants that have health-promoting properties, such as antioxidants, flavonoids, and carotenoids. They are not considered essential nutrients but have been shown to have beneficial effects on health.

"Phytochemicals are naturally occurring compounds in plants that have health-promoting properties, such as antioxidants, flavonoids, and carotenoids."

THE ROLE OF MICRONUTRIENTS AND PHYTOCHEMICALS IN WHOLE-FOODS

Whole-foods, such as fruits, vegetables, whole grains, legumes, and nuts, are typically high in micronutrients and phytochemicals. These essential nutrients play critical roles in maintaining good health and preventing chronic diseases.

Micronutrients, such as vitamins and minerals, are essential for many of the body's functions. They help to maintain a healthy immune system, support proper growth and development, protect against oxidative stress and inflammation, and promote overall well-being. For example, vitamin C supports a healthy immune system, vitamin D helps to regulate calcium and phosphorus metabolism, and iron supports the production of hemoglobin which helps to carry oxygen in the blood.

Phytochemicals are naturally occurring compounds found in plants that have health-promoting properties. They are not essential nutrients but have been shown to have beneficial effects on health.

Phytochemicals have anti-inflammatory and antioxidant effects, and may help to reduce the risk of chronic diseases such as cancer and heart disease. For example, flavonoids are a type of phytochemical that have been shown to have anti-inflammatory properties, and carotenoids are a type of phytochemical that have been shown to have antioxidant properties.

THE IMPACT OF PROCESSING ON NUTRIENT DENSITY

The impact of processing on nutrient density refers to the changes in the nutritional value of foods that occur during food processing. Processing methods such as cooking, canning, freezing, and drying can alter the nutrient content of foods. The extent of nutrient loss depends on the specific processing method and the food being processed.

Processing can lead to a loss of micronutrients such as vitamins and minerals. For example, vitamin C is sensitive to heat and can be lost during cooking, and vitamin A is sensitive to light and can be lost during storage. Processing can also lead to a loss of phytochemicals, which are known for their health-promoting properties. Additionally, processing can lead to the addition of unhealthy ingredients such as added sugars, sodium, and unhealthy fats.

Processed foods, such as packaged snacks and frozen dinners, often have lower nutrient density than whole foods, as they are often high in calories and low in essential vitamins, minerals, and phytochemicals.

Processed foods are often fortified with synthetic vitamins and minerals, but they can't replace the natural micronutrients and phytochemicals that are present in whole foods.

Whole-foods are generally considered to be more nutritious than processed foods, as they retain most of their natural micronutrients and phytochemicals. Eating a diet rich in whole-foods can help to ensure that you're getting the most nutritious bang for your buck.

CHAPTER TWO

Building a Nutrient-Dense Diet

This chapter covers building a nutrient-dense diet. It includes principles of including whole-grains, fruits, vegetables, legumes, nuts, and seeds in daily meals, the role of healthy fats and proteins, importance of diversity, seasonal and local eating, fermented foods and cooking methods on preserving nutrient density. It helps readers to create a diet tailored to their individual needs for optimal health through nutrient-dense eating.

THE IMPORTANCE OF A PLANT-BASED DIET

Introducing a plant-based diet, which emphasizes whole, unprocessed plant foods such as fruits, vegetables, whole grains, legumes, nuts, and seeds, can have a profound impact on one's health and well-being. The benefits of a plant-based diet are numerous, as it is naturally low in saturated fat and cholesterol, and high in fiber, antioxidants, and phytochemicals. This nutritional profile has been shown to reduce the risk of chronic illnesses such as coronary heart disease, diabetes, and certain cancers by lowering inflammation in the body and improving overall health.

Not only is a plant-based diet beneficial for overall health, it also can aid in weight management. Plant-based diets are naturally lower in calories and higher in fiber, making it a great option for weight management. Another added benefit of a plant-based diet is its positive impact on the environment, requiring fewer resources to produce and generating less greenhouse gas emissions.

But the benefits of a plant-based diet aren't limited to just health and environmental impact, it also offers a wide variety of delicious and flavorful foods to be enjoyed. It can also be easily adapted to different cultural and personal preferences.

Studies have shown that plant-based diets are associated with lower rates of depression, anxiety and stress. This may be due to the high intake of antioxidants and anti-inflammatory compounds found in fruits, vegetables, whole grains and legumes, which can protect the brain from damage and improve brain function.

Another benefit of a plant-based diet is that it can improve gut health. Plant-based diets are high in fiber, which helps to feed the beneficial bacteria in the gut and promote a healthy gut microbiome.

This can lead to improved digestion, regular bowel movements and a reduction in inflammation throughout the body. One of the most important things to keep in mind when transitioning to a plant-based diet is to make sure to get enough protein. Plant-based sources of protein such as beans, lentils, tofu, and tempeh can easily provide enough protein to meet the body's needs.

Choosing a plant-based diet can seem daunting, but it doesn't have to be. It's about making a commitment to try new foods, experimenting with different recipes and being open to incorporating more plant-based foods into your diet. Small, incremental changes can lead to big benefits in the long run. lant-based diet that will leave you feeling healthier and happier.

CHOOSING NUTRIENT-DENSE FOODS FOR OPTIMAL HEALTH

Aside to the traditional nutrient-dense foods like leafy greens and berries, there are also some lesser-known options that pack a powerful nutritional punch. For example, sea vegetables like nori, dulse, and kelp are packed with minerals like iodine and iron, which are essential for healthy thyroid function and red blood cell production. They also contain high levels of antioxidants, which can help to protect against chronic diseases like cancer and heart disease.

Another exciting option for nutrient-dense eating is fermented foods. Foods like kimchi, sauerkraut, and kefir are excellent sources of probiotics, which can help to improve gut health and boost the immune system. They also tend to be rich in enzymes and other beneficial compounds that can aid in digestion and nutrient absorption.

Another way to boost the nutrient density of your diet is by incorporating more nuts and seeds. Foods like chia seeds, flax seeds, and hemp seeds are rich in essential fatty acids, protein, and minerals like magnesium and zinc. Nuts like almonds, walnuts, and pistachios also contain healthy fats, protein, and a variety of micronutrients.

Lastly, incorporating more herbs and spices into your diet can be a great way to boost nutrient density. Turmeric, ginger, and cinnamon are all known for their anti-inflammatory and antioxidant properties and can be added to a variety of dishes to boost their nutritional value. With a little experimentation and creativity, eating a nutrient-dense diet can be fun, delicious, and easy to maintain.

"fermented foods. Foods like kimchi, sauerkraut, and kefir are excellent sources of probiotics, which can help to improve gut health and boost the immune system."

MEAL PLANNING AND PREPARATION STRATEGIES FOR A NUTRIENT-DENSE DIET

Life can get too busy and somethings overwhelming for most, making the adaptation of a nutrient-dense diet abit challenging to maintain without proper planning and preparation. Here are some of the strategies to employ.

Meal Planning

These are some meal planning strategies to note:

☐ Plan your meals in advance, taking into consideration the nutrient density of each food. This means choosing foods that are high in vitamins, minerals, and phytochemicals, while being low in added sugars, saturated fats, and processed ingredients.

☐ Use a food diary to keep track of the nutrients you are consuming. This can help you identify any deficiencies and make adjustments to your diet accordingly.

☐ Make a grocery list and stick to it to avoid impulse buys. This will help you to stay on track and ensure that you have all the necessary ingredients on hand to make healthy meals.

☐ Try to incorporate a variety of different foods and food groups into your diet. Eating a wide range of fruits, vegetables, whole grains, legumes, nuts, and seeds will ensure that you are getting a balance of all the essential nutrients your body needs.

Meal Preparation

☐ Wash and chop vegetables in advance to make them easy to grab and go. This makes it convenient to add them to meals throughout the week.

☐ Cook extra food and freeze it for later. This is a great way to have healthy meals on hand when you don't have time to cook from scratch.

☐ Make sure you have healthy snacks on hand like raw veggies, nuts, and seeds. This will help to keep you from reaching for less nutritious options.

☐ Try to cook at home as much as possible so you can control the ingredients and the cooking method. This will help you to ensure that you are eating a nutrient-dense diet and not consuming unnecessary calories, sodium, and added sugars.

Portion Control

☐ Be mindful of portion sizes and eat until you are satisfied, not until you are full. Eating too much can lead to weight gain and other health issues.

- ⏴ Use smaller plates to help you control portions. This will help to ensure that you are not eating more than you need.

- ⏴ Avoid eating in front of the television or computer. This can lead to overeating and not paying attention to your body's signals of fullness.

- ⏴ Take your time to savor your food and enjoy the flavors. Eating slowly can help you to feel full faster and eat less.

Maintaining a nutrient-dense diet is crucial for optimal health, and meal planning and preparation strategies play a significant role in achieving this. One effective strategy is to focus on whole, unprocessed foods such as fruits, vegetables, whole grains, legumes, nuts, and seeds. These foods provide a wide range of essential vitamins, minerals, and phytochemicals that our bodies need.

Another important strategy is to choose cooking methods that preserve the nutrient density of foods. This includes techniques like steaming, baking, and sautéing. On the other hand, high-heat methods like frying can strip foods of their valuable nutrients, so it's best to avoid them.

Summary

Food preparation is equally crucial to make it easy to eat nutrient-dense foods throughout the day. For example, prepping and portioning out snacks like cut-up fruits and vegetables can make it easy to grab a healthy snack when you're on the go. Similarly, preparing and portioning out meals in advance can make it easy to stick to a nutrient-dense diet even when you're short on time.

☐ Focusing on whole, unprocessed foods

☐ Utilizing cooking methods that preserve nutrient density

☐ Preparing and portioning out meals and snacks in advance

☐ Avoiding high-heat cooking methods.

CHAPTER THREE

Whole-Foods and Disease Prevention

This chapter explores the mechanisms by which specific whole-foods and food groups can improve biomarkers and reduce the risk of disease, providing practical advice on how to incorporate these foods into a daily routine.

THE LINK BETWEEN WHOLE-FOODS AND CHRONIC DISEASE PREVENTION

The relationship between whole-foods and chronic disease prevention is a topic of increasing interest among health experts. Whole-foods, such as fruits, vegetables, whole grains, legumes, nuts, and seeds, are considered to be the key players in preventing chronic diseases. These foods are nutrient-dense, high in fiber, low in added sugars, saturated fats, and processed ingredients, and provide a plethora of health benefits.

A diet rich in fruits and vegetables is associated with a reduced risk of heart disease, stroke, and certain types of cancer. Whole grains, such as oats, quinoa, and brown rice, have been linked to a lower risk of type 2 diabetes and heart disease. Legumes, such as black beans, lentils, and chickpeas, are high in protein and have been shown to lower cholesterol and blood pressure. Nuts and seeds, such as almonds and flaxseeds, are a good source of healthy fats and have been linked to a lower risk of heart disease.

Eating a diet rich in whole-foods can also help to maintain a healthy weight. Whole-foods are generally low in calories, high in fiber, and nutrient-dense, which can help to keep you feeling full and satisfied. This can lead to eating less and ultimately, weight loss. They also promote healthy digestion, support a strong immune system, and improve cognitive function.

Other factors such as Physical exercise, stress reduction, and hereditary characteristics also play a role. However, incorporating a diet rich in whole-foods can provide a strong foundation for overall health and well-being, and it can also serve as a protective measure against chronic diseases.

One of the ways to implement a whole-foods diet is to focus on a variety of colorful fruits and vegetables. Each color represents a different group of phytochemicals that provide unique health benefits. For example, dark leafy greens are high in vitamin K which is important for bone health, while red fruits and vegetables are high in lycopene which is known to reduce the risk of heart disease.

It's also important to include a variety of plant-based protein sources in your diet such as legumes, nuts, and seeds. Eating a variety of plant-based protein sources can also help to reduce the risk of chronic diseases such as heart disease.

Integrating a variety of whole-foods in your diet is not only beneficial for chronic disease prevention, but it can also provide a wide range of health benefits. The key is to eat a variety of whole-foods and to enjoy them in their natural state as much as possible. By doing so, you can ensure that you're getting all the essential nutrients your body needs to thrive.

THE IMPACT OF WHOLE-FOODS ON CARDIOVASCULAR HEALTH

The impact of whole-foods on cardiovascular health is significant. Whole-foods, such as fruits, vegetables, whole grains, legumes, nuts, and seeds, are rich in nutrients that are essential for maintaining a healthy heart. These foods are high in fiber, vitamins, and minerals, and are low in added sugars, saturated fats, and processed ingredients, which can contribute to the development of cardiovascular disease.

Eating a diet rich in fruits and vegetables can lower the likelihood of developing heart disease. These foods are high in antioxidants, such as vitamins C and E, which help to protect the heart from damage caused by free radicals. They are also high in potassium, which can help to lower blood pressure, and folate, which can reduce the risk of heart disease.

Whole grains have also been linked to a lower risk of heart disease. They are high in fiber, which can help to lower cholesterol and blood pressure, and contain antioxidants, such as vitamin E, that protect the heart. Legumes, such as beans, lentils, and peas, are also high in fiber and have been shown to lower cholesterol and blood pressure.

Nuts and seeds are a good source of healthy fats, such as omega-3 fatty acids, which can help to reduce inflammation and lower the risk of heart disease. They also contain antioxidants and minerals, such as magnesium and potassium, that are essential for maintaining a healthy heart.

WHOLE-FOODS AND CANCER PREVENTION

Research has shown that consuming a diet high in whole-foods, such as fruits, vegetables, whole grains, legumes, nuts, and seeds, can significantly reduce the risk of certain types of cancer.

Fruits and vegetables, in particular, are rich in antioxidants and phytochemicals that can help to neutralize harmful free radicals and protect against DNA damage. For example, cruciferous vegetables like broccoli, cauliflower, and Brussels sprouts contain compounds called glucosinolates, which have been shown to have anti-cancer properties. Similarly, tomatoes are a rich source of lycopene, a carotenoid that has been linked to a lower risk of prostate cancer.

Whole grains, legumes, and nuts are also important for cancer prevention. Whole grains, such as oats, barley, and quinoa, are high in fiber and have been linked to a lower risk of colorectal cancer. Legumes, like beans, lentils, and peas, are rich in protein, fiber, and phytochemicals that can help to lower the risk of breast cancer. Nuts, such as almonds, walnuts, and pecans, are a good source of healthy fats and have been associated with a lower risk of breast cancer.

It is important to note that cancer is a complex disease that can be influenced by a variety of factors, including genetics, lifestyle, and environment. However, adopting a diet rich in whole-foods is an essential step towards cancer prevention and overall health. Eating a variety of nutrient-dense foods on a regular basis can help to provide the body with the essential nutrients it needs to function properly and protect against disease.

CHAPTER FOUR

Whole-Foods and Longevity

This chapter explores the specific nutrients and phytochemicals found in whole-foods that have been linked to longevity and age-related disease prevention, as well as practical tips for incorporating more whole-foods into one's diet for optimal health and well-being as we age.

THE ROLE OF WHOLE-FOODS IN AGING AND LONGEVITY

Eating a diet rich in whole-foods, such as fruits, vegetables, whole grains, legumes, nuts, and seeds, has been linked to better health outcomes and a longer life span. One of the key ways that whole-foods support longevity is through their anti-inflammatory properties. Chronic inflammation has been linked to a host of age-related diseases, including heart disease, cancer, and Alzheimer's. Whole-foods, particularly fruits and vegetables, are rich in antioxidants and phytochemicals that help to combat inflammation in the body.

Another way that whole-foods support longevity is through their ability to promote healthy digestion and a strong immune system. A diet rich in fiber and other nutrients found in whole-foods can help to keep the gut microbiome in balance, which is essential for maintaining overall health. A healthy gut microbiome has been linked to a lower risk of chronic diseases, including cancer and heart disease.

In addition to their anti-inflammatory properties and support for healthy digestion, whole-foods also play a role in maintaining a healthy weight. Eating a diet rich in whole-foods can help to reduce the risk of obesity, which is a major risk factor for a host of age-related diseases. All in all, the role of whole-foods in aging and longevity is multifaceted. Adopting a whole-foods diet can not only help to reduce the risk of age-related diseases, but also promote overall health and well-being.

THE IMPACT OF A NUTRIENT-DENSE DIET ON COGNITIVE FUNCTION AND BRAIN HEALTH

Adopting a nutrient-dense diet, can have a significant impact on cognitive function and brain health. These foods are rich in essential nutrients, including antioxidants, vitamins, and minerals, that are vital for optimal brain function.

Studies have shown that consuming a diet high in fruits and vegetables, particularly leafy greens, is associated with a lower risk of cognitive decline and a reduced risk of developing Alzheimer's disease. The antioxidants and anti-inflammatory compounds found in these foods can help to protect the brain from damage caused by free radicals and inflammation.

Whole grains have also been shown to have a positive impact on cognitive function. Whole grains, such as oats and quinoa, are rich in B-vitamins and antioxidants, which are essential for maintaining brain health. They also provide the brain with a steady supply of energy, which can help to improve cognitive function and concentration.

Omega-3 fatty acids, found in fatty fish, nuts and seeds, can also play an important role in maintaining brain health. These essential fats are important for the development and function of the brain, and have been shown to improve memory and cognitive function.

Incorporating whole food into your eat habits can help to protect the brain from damage, improve cognitive function and concentration, and reduce the risk of cognitive decline and age-related diseases

WHOLE-FOODS AND PHYSICAL PERFORMANCE

Eating a diet rich in whole-foods can have a significant impact on physical performance. Whole-foods, provide the body with the essential nutrients it needs to function properly which can protect the body against inflammation and cellular damage.

Consuming a diet high in whole-foods can improve muscle and bone health, leading to increased strength and endurance. Whole grains, for example, provide a good source of carbohydrates, which are the primary fuel for the body during physical activity. Legumes, such as beans and lentils, are high in protein, which is essential for building and repairing muscle tissue. Nuts and seeds, meanwhile, are a great source of healthy fats, which can help to maintain joint health and reduce inflammation.

Eating a diet rich in whole-foods can also improve cardiovascular health, which is crucial for physical performance. Whole-foods are low in saturated fats and high in fiber, which can help to lower cholesterol and blood pressure. This can lead to improved blood flow, which can in turn lead to better oxygen delivery to the muscles during physical activity. They can also help to maintain a healthy weight, which is important for physical performance.

CHAPTER FIVE

Whole-Foods and the Environment

This chapter explores the connection between our food choices and issues such as climate change, deforestation, and water scarcity, and how a whole-foods diet can play a critical role in building a more sustainable food system, , as well as how a shift towards whole-foods can help to mitigate the negative effects of industrial agriculture and factory   farming.

THE ENVIRONMENTAL IMPACT OF A NUTRIENT-DENSE, PLANT-BASED DIET

Nutrient-dense, plant-based diet also has a positive impact on the environment. A diet rich in fruits, vegetables, whole grains, legumes, nuts, and seeds requires less land, water, and other resources to produce compared to a diet high in animal products.

Animal agriculture is a leading cause of deforestation, water and air pollution, and greenhouse gas emissions. Livestock is responsible for 14.5% of global greenhouse gas emissions and is a major contributor to deforestation, as land is cleared for grazing and feed crops. Animal agriculture also requires large amounts of water and is a leading cause of water pollution.

On the other hand, plant-based foods are much more sustainable to produce. They require less land and water, and have a lower carbon footprint. Eating a diet rich in whole-foods can also lead to less food waste, as these foods are typically fresher and have a longer shelf life.

In summary, a nutrient-dense, plant-based diet not only benefits personal health, but it also helps to reduce the environmental impact of the food system. Adopting a diet rich in whole-foods is a step towards a more sustainable

"Choosing seasonal and local foods not only supports the environment, but also ensures optimal freshness and nutrient content.."

food system and a healthier planet.

STRATEGIES FOR REDUCING YOUR ENVIRONMENTAL FOOTPRINT THROUGH WHOLE-FOODS

Nutrient-dense, plant-based diet not only has positive effects on personal health, but also on the environment. Animal farming is a primary factor contributing to the emission of greenhouse gases, air and water contamination, as well as deforestation.. A diet rich in fruits, vegetables, whole grains, and legumes requires less land, water, and other resources to produce compared to a diet high in animal products.

To reduce your environmental footprint through whole-foods, consider implementing the following strategies:

- ⬜ Buy local and seasonal produce to reduce the carbon emissions associated with transportation and to support your community's farmers.

- ⬜ Choose organic foods to support sustainable farming practices and reduce the use of harmful pesticides and fertilizers.

- ⬜ Incorporate plant-based proteins such as beans, lentils, and tofu in place of animal products.

- ⬜ Use reusable containers and bags when shopping for groceries to reduce waste.

- ⬜ Grow your own fruits and vegetables in a backyard or community garden.

⏥ Support sustainable fishing practices by choosing seafood that is certified by organizations such as the Marine Stewardship Council.

⏥ Educate yourself about the environmental impact of the foods you are consuming and make informed choices.

By incorporating these strategies, you can make a significant impact on reducing your environmental footprint and promoting sustainability through your dietary choices.

ECONOMIC IMPACT OF THE CURRENT FOOD SYSTEM AND THE POTENTIAL BENEFITS

The current food system, which relies heavily on processed and packaged foods, has a significant economic impact. According to data from the USDA, Americans spent an estimated $1.7 trillion on food in 2019, with nearly 60% of that spending going towards processed and packaged foods. In contrast, only 10% of food spending went towards fruits and vegetables, which are essential components of a whole-foods diet.

This disproportionate spending on processed and packaged foods is due in part to the fact that they are often cheaper and more accessible than fresh, whole foods. However, there are hidden costs associated with this type of food system. For example, the long-term health effects of a diet high in processed and packaged foods can lead to chronic diseases such as heart disease, type 2 diabetes, and obesity, which can result in significant healthcare costs.

A shift towards a whole-foods diet has the potential to not only improve individual health but also have positive economic impacts on society as a whole. By supporting local farmers and producers, consumers can help create a more sustainable food system that prioritizes fresh, seasonal, and nutrient-dense foods.

Additionally, a whole-foods diet can help reduce healthcare costs associated with chronic diseases. According to a study published in the Journal of Hunger & Environmental Nutrition, increasing fruit and vegetable intake by just one serving per day could save $5 billion annually in healthcare costs.

Moreover, supporting local and regional food systems can create jobs and stimulate economic growth in communities. According to the USDA, small farms are responsible for creating nearly 50% of all jobs in the U.S. food system. The economic impact of our current food system extends beyond the cost of food at the grocery store.

CHAPTER SIX

Whole-Foods and Social Justice

This chapter explores the intersection of food systems and societal inequalities. It delves into how access to nutrient-dense, whole foods is not equitable for all individuals and communities and the impact this has on health outcomes. Additionally, it examines the economic and political factors that contribute to these inequalities and discusses ways to promote food justice through whole-foods.

THE IMPACT OF FOOD SYSTEMS ON SOCIAL JUSTICE

The impact of food systems on social justice is a complex and multi-faceted issue that requires a critical examination of the ways in which our food is grown, processed, distributed, and consumed. At its core, social justice in the food system is about ensuring that all individuals have equal access to healthy, culturally appropriate, and sustainable food.

One major aspect of food systems and social justice is the way in which food is grown and produced. Industrial agriculture, for example, has been shown to disproportionately harm low-income communities and communities of color by exposing them to harmful pesticides and other chemicals. Additionally, the industrialization of agriculture has led to the displacement of small farmers and the consolidation of farmland into the hands of a few large corporations.

An important aspect of food systems and social justice is access to healthy food. Low-income communities and communities of color are often located in "food deserts," areas with limited access to fresh fruits and vegetables and a disproportionate number of fast food and convenience stores. These communities often have higher rates of diet-related chronic diseases as a result.

Addressing social justice in the food system requires a holistic approach that includes everything from fair labor practices for farm workers to policies that promote local and sustainable food systems. Ultimately, a just and equitable food system is one in which all people have the ability to access nutritious, culturally appropriate food that is grown and produced in a way that is sustainable for both people and the planet.

STRATEGIES FOR SUPPORTING FAIR AND EQUITABLE FOOD SYSTEMS THROUGH WHOLE-FOODS

The current industrial food system often prioritizes profit over people and the planet, resulting in injustices such as poverty, food insecurity, and environmental degradation.

One way to support fair and equitable food systems through whole-foods is by choosing to buy from local and organic farmers. This helps to support small-scale farmers and reduce the carbon footprint associated with long-distance transportation of food. Additionally, choosing to buy from farmers who prioritize fair labor practices and pay their workers a living wage can help to promote social justice within the food system.

Local and seasonal foods vary by region and are dependent on climate and growing conditions. Here are some examples of local and seasonal foods that are commonly available in different regions:

- Northeast: Apples, pumpkins, squash, sweet potatoes, beets, carrots, cabbage, kale, spinach, and cranberries.

- ☐ Midwest: Corn, tomatoes, zucchini, green beans, peaches, plums, cherries, raspberries, and blueberries.

- ☐ Southeast: Okra, collard greens, sweet potatoes, watermelon, peaches, strawberries, and pecans.

- ☐ Southwest: Peppers, tomatoes, corn, avocados, melons, and citrus fruits.

- ☐ Northwest: Apples, pears, berries, cherries, mushrooms, kale, and squash.

Another strategy is to support food sovereignty, which is the right of people to healthy and culturally appropriate food produced through ecologically sound and sustainable methods. This can be done by supporting community gardens and local food systems, as well as advocating for policies that prioritize small-scale and sustainable agriculture.

Lastly, it is important to be mindful of the impact of our food choices on indigenous people and traditional farming practices. Supporting indigenous-led initiatives and traditional farming practices can help to preserve cultural heritage and promote food sovereignty. By making conscious choices about the food we consume and where it comes from, we have the power to support fair and equitable food systems.

Conclusion

WHOLE-FOODS AND PHYSICAL PERFORMANCE

Eating a diet rich in whole-foods can have a significant impact on physical performance. Whole-food provide the body with the essential nutrients it needs to function properly, which can protect the body against inflammation and cellular damage.

Consuming a diet high in whole-foods can improve muscle and bone health, leading to increased strength and endurance. Whole grains, for example, provide a good source of carbohydrates, which are the primary fuel for the body during physical activity. Legumes, such as beans and lentils, are high in protein, which is essential for building and repairing muscle tissue. Nuts and seeds, meanwhile, are a great source of healthy fats, which can help to maintain joint health and reduce inflammation.

Eating a diet rich in whole-foods can also improve cardiovascular health, which is crucial for physical performance. Whole-foods are low in saturated fats and high in fiber, which can help to lower cholesterol and blood pressure. This can lead to improved blood flow, which can in turn lead to better oxygen delivery to the muscles during physical activity. They can also help to maintain a healthy weight, which is important for physical performance

Individuals who have adopted a whole-foods diet have reported numerous positive impacts on their health. Many have claimed to have increased energy levels, improved digestion, better sleep, and weight loss.

For instance, some have reported improved mental clarity and reduced brain fog, leading to increased productivity and a sense of overall well-being. Others have seen a significant reduction in their blood pressure, cholesterol levels, and blood sugar, leading to better management of chronic diseases such as diabetes and heart disease.

Furthermore, many individuals have noticed a positive change in their skin, with acne and other skin conditions clearing up. Some have also reported a reduction in joint pain, inflammation, and arthritis symptoms.

TRANSITIONING TO A WHOLE-FOODS DIET

Meal Planning and Grocery shopping.

As someone who has personally made the switch, I know firsthand how challenging it can be to navigate this new way of eating. But with a bit of planning and preparation, it is entirely possible to make the transition and stick with it long-term.

Here are some meal planning and grocery shopping tips that have helped me on my whole-foods journey:

- ☐ Plan your meals for the week ahead: Taking the time to plan out your meals for the week can help you avoid last-minute decisions that could lead you back to unhealthy eating habits. Start by writing down what you plan to eat for breakfast, lunch, and dinner each day. Then make a grocery list of the ingredients you'll need.

- ☐ Shop at your local farmers' market: One of the best ways to find local, seasonal produce is by shopping at your local farmers' market. Not only will you be supporting local farmers, but you'll also have access to fresh, in-season produce that is often more flavorful and nutrient-dense than what you'll find at the supermarket.

- ☐ Buy in bulk: Buying in bulk is an excellent way to save money and reduce waste. Look for items like nuts, seeds, grains, and legumes that you can buy in larger quantities and store in airtight containers. This will also help you avoid last-minute trips to the store when you run out of a particular ingredient.

- ☐ Stick to your grocery list: It's easy to get sidetracked when you're shopping for groceries, but sticking to your list can help you avoid impulse buys that could derail your healthy eating goals. Focus on buying whole, nutrient-dense foods and avoid processed foods and snacks.

▢ Prep ahead of time: Taking a few hours each week to prep ahead can save you time and stress during the week. Cook a batch of brown rice or quinoa, chop up veggies for salads and snacks, and roast a tray of sweet potatoes or other root vegetables. This will make it easier to throw together healthy meals and snacks when you're short on time.

Remember, transitioning to a whole-foods diet is a journey, and it's okay to make mistakes along the way. Don't be too hard on yourself if you slip up and indulge in a processed snack or meal. Just focus on getting back on track and making small, sustainable changes over time.

Food culture has evolved over time, shaped by various factors such as geography, climate, agriculture, religion, and social customs. Different regions and cultures have developed unique food traditions and culinary practices, often reflecting their natural resources, beliefs, and values. For example, Mediterranean cuisine is known for its abundant use of fresh fruits, vegetables, legumes, and olive oil, while Japanese cuisine emphasizes simplicity, balance, and seasonality.

However, the advent of industrialization, urbanization, and globalization has transformed the way we produce, distribute, and consume food. The modern food system is characterized by large-scale farming, intensive animal agriculture, food processing and packaging, long-distance transportation, and retail consolidation. While these changes have led to greater efficiency, affordability, and convenience, they have also resulted in a number of challenges and consequences.

One of the main issues with the current food system is the prevalence of highly processed, calorie-dense, nutrient-poor foods, which are often marketed and sold as cheap and convenient options. These foods are often high in added sugars, unhealthy fats, and sodium, and contribute to the rising rates of obesity, diabetes, heart disease, and other chronic health conditions.

In addition, the industrialization of food production has led to a loss of biodiversity, soil degradation, water pollution, and greenhouse gas emissions, which have negative impacts on both the environment and human health. Moreover, the concentration of food production and distribution in the hands of a few large corporations has resulted in economic inequalities and exploitation of workers, particularly in developing countries.

Despite these challenges, there has been a growing movement towards sustainable and healthy food systems, which prioritize local and seasonal foods, small-scale and diversified agriculture, regenerative farming practices, and equitable food access. The shift towards whole-foods and nutrient-dense eating is a key aspect of this movement, as it promotes the consumption of minimally processed, whole, and fresh foods that are rich in vitamins, minerals, fiber, and phytonutrients.

By understanding the history of food culture and how it relates to the current food system, we can better appreciate the value of whole-foods and the need for a more sustainable and equitable food future.

Several case studies and research have been conducted on specific populations or communities that have benefited from a whole-foods diet. Here are a few examples:

Blue Zones: The Blue Zones are regions around the world where people tend to live longer and healthier lives. These regions include Okinawa, Japan; Sardinia, Italy; Nicoya, Costa Rica; Icaria, Greece; and Loma Linda, California. Researchers have found that these populations consume a whole-foods diet that is rich in vegetables, fruits, whole grains, and legumes, and low in processed foods and animal products.

African Americans: African Americans have a higher risk of chronic diseases such as diabetes, heart disease, and obesity. However, research has shown that adopting a whole-foods diet can significantly reduce the risk of these diseases. A study conducted by the Physicians Committee for Responsible Medicine found that African Americans who switched to a whole-foods, plant-based diet experienced significant reductions in blood pressure, cholesterol levels, and weight.

Indigenous Communities: Indigenous communities around the world have traditionally consumed whole-foods diets that are rich in local and seasonal fruits, vegetables, and grains. However, as these communities have been exposed to western diets, they have experienced a rise in chronic diseases. Researchers have found that promoting the consumption of traditional whole-foods diets can help prevent and manage chronic diseases in these communities.

Children: Children who consume whole-foods diets have been found to have better health outcomes, including lower rates of obesity and chronic diseases. A study published in the American Journal of Clinical Nutrition found that children who consumed a diet rich in fruits, vegetables, and whole grains had lower levels of inflammation in their bodies, which is a risk factor for chronic diseases. Additionally, a study published in the Journal of School Health found that children who were offered whole-foods options in school cafeterias were more likely to choose them and consume them.

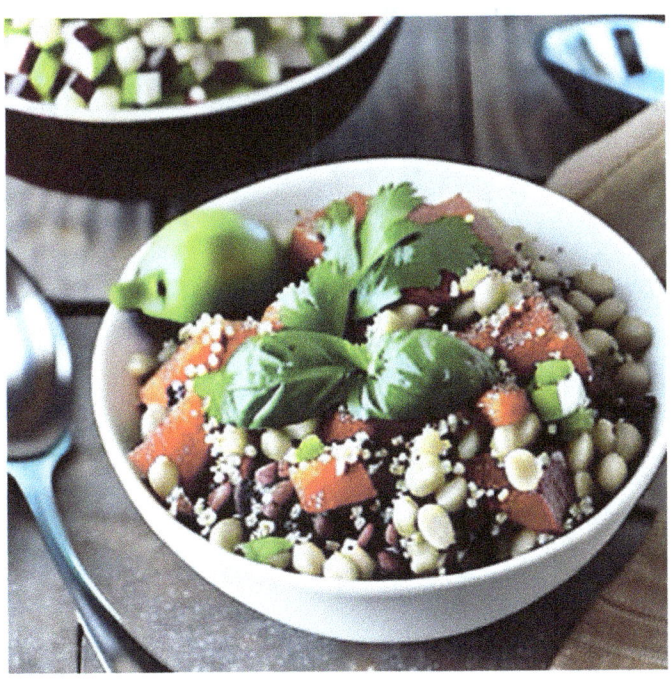

Appendix: Recipes and Meal Plans

QUINOA AND BLACK BEAN SALAD:

Ingredents

1 cup cooked quinoa

1 can black beans, rinsed and drained

1 red bell pepper, diced

1/2 red onion, diced

1/4 cup cilantro, chopped

1 lime, juiced

1 tablespoon olive oil

Salt and pepper, to taste.

Preparation

Mix all ingredients together in a large bowl and season with salt and pepper to taste. Serve chilled or at room temperature.

Whole Grain Pasta with Spinach and Tomatoes:

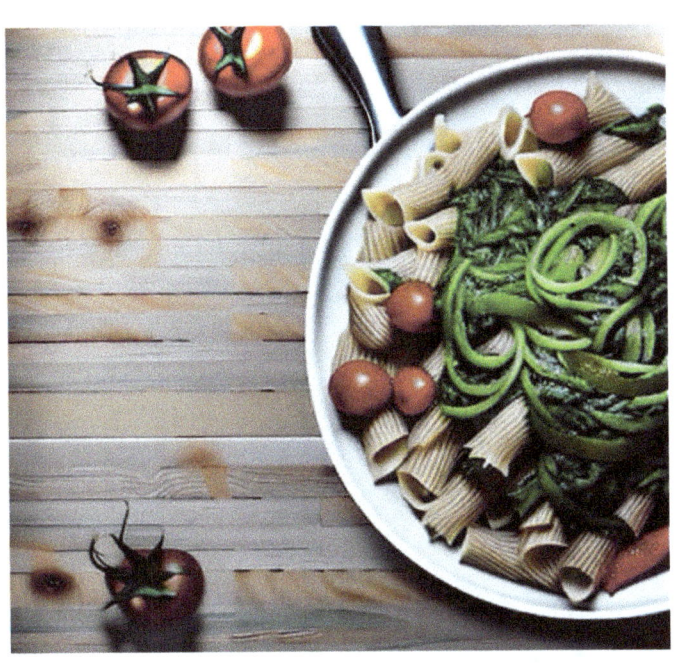

Ingredients

8 oz whole grain pasta

2 cups spinach

1 cup cherry tomatoes, halved

2 cloves garlic, minced

2 tablespoons olive oil

Salt and pepper, to taste

Cook pasta according to package instructions. In a separate pan, sauté garlic in olive oil over medium heat. Add spinach and tomatoes and cook until wilted. Toss with cooked pasta and season with salt and pepper to taste.

SWEET POTATO AND BLACK BEAN ENCHILADAS:

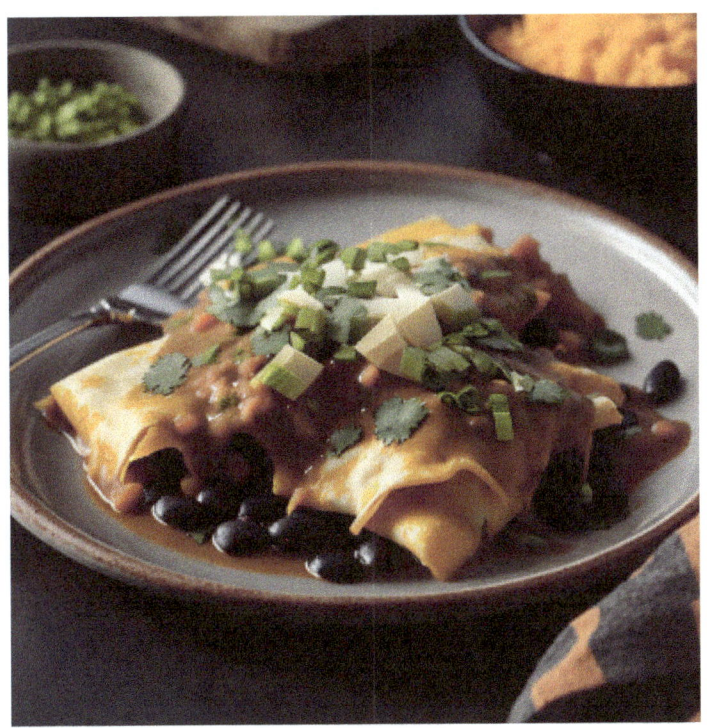

Ingredents

8 whole wheat tortillas

1 sweet potato, peeled and diced

1 can black beans, rinsed and drained

1/2 cup diced onion

1/2 cup diced bell pepper

1 cup enchilada sauce

1/2 cup shredded cheddar cheese

Salt and pepper, to taste

Preheat oven to 375 degrees. In a pan, sauté sweet potato, black beans, onion, and bell pepper until tender. Mix in enchilada sauce and season with salt and pepper to taste. Spread a spoonful of mixture on each tortilla and roll up. Place enchiladas in a baking dish and top with shredded cheese. Bake for 15-20 minutes or until cheese is melted and bubbly.

MEAL PLAN

Monday:
Breakfast: Whole grain toast with avocado and scrambled eggs

Lunch: Quinoa and black bean salad

Dinner: Whole grain pasta with spinach and tomatoes

Tuesday:
Breakfast: Oatmeal with berries and chopped nuts

Lunch: Whole grain sandwich with hummus, vegetables, and avocado

Dinner: Sweet potato and black bean enchiladas

Wednesday:
Breakfast: Smoothie bowl with frozen berries, spinach, and Greek yogurt

Lunch: Whole grain salad with mixed greens, vegetables, and a vinaigrette dressing

Dinner: Baked fish with a whole grain side and steamed vegetables

Thursday:
Breakfast: Whole grain pancakes with fresh fruit

Lunch: Whole grain wrap with grilled vegetables and a tahini sauce

Dinner: Lentil and vegetable curry with a whole grain side.

Friday:

Breakfast: Whole grain English muffin with peanut butter and banana

Lunch: Whole grain sushi rolls with mixed vegetables and a soy-ginger dipping sauce

Dinner: Whole grain pizzas with a variety of vegetable toppings

Saturday:

Breakfast: Whole grain waffles with fresh fruit and maple syrup

Lunch: Whole grain soup with mixed vegetables and a whole grain roll

Dinner: Whole grain stir-fry with mixed vegetables and a choice of protein (tofu, chicken, or shrimp)

Sunday:

Breakfast: Whole grain French toast with fresh fruit and syrup

Lunch: Whole grain bowl with mixed greens, vegetables, and a choice of protein (chickpeas, chicken, or tofu)

Dinner: Whole grain lasagna with mixed vegetables and a choice of protein (tofu, chicken, or ground turkey)

Appendix A: Recipes and Meal Plans

Whole-Foods Breakfast Ideas

- ? Avocado toast with a fried egg and tomato

- ? Oatmeal with fresh berries, chopped nuts, and a drizzle of honey

- ? Smoothie bowl made with frozen fruit, spinach, and Greek yogurt

- ? Whole-grain waffles topped with fresh fruit and a drizzle of maple syrup

- ? Veggie and cheese omelette

Whole-Foods Lunch Ideas

- ? Whole-grain wrap filled with hummus, veggies, and grilled chicken

- Lentil soup with a side salad of mixed greens

- Quinoa bowl with roasted veggies, black beans, and avocado

- Whole-grain pasta with a homemade tomato sauce, topped with grated Parmesan cheese

- Whole-grain pizza with a variety of veggies and mozzarella cheese

Whole-Foods Dinner Ideas

- Grilled chicken breast with a side of roasted sweet potatoes and steamed broccoli

- Whole-grain risotto with sautéed vegetables and shrimp

- Whole-grain stir-fry with a variety of veggies, tofu, and a homemade sauce

- Whole-grain lasagna with a homemade meat or vegetable sauce

- Whole-grain tacos filled with seasoned ground beef or chicken, topped with lettuce, cheese, and salsa

Whole-Foods Snack Ideas

- Fresh fruit with a side of yogurt

- Homemade trail mix with a variety of nuts and dried fruit

- Whole-grain crackers with hummus or avocado spread

- Whole-grain pita chips with a side of homemade salsa

- Apple slices with a drizzle of peanut butter

Whole-Foods Meal Plan

Monday:

Breakfast: Avocado toast with a fried egg and tomato

Lunch: Whole-grain wrap filled with hummus, veggies, and grilled chicken

Dinner: Grilled chicken breast with a side of roasted sweet potatoes and steamed broccoli

Tuesday:

Breakfast: Oatmeal with fresh berries, chopped nuts, and a drizzle of honey

Lunch: Lentil soup with a side salad of mixed greens

Dinner: Whole-grain risotto with sautéed vegetables and shrimp

Wednesday:

Breakfast: Smoothie bowl made with frozen fruit, spinach, and Greek yogurt

Lunch: Quinoa bowl with roasted veggies, black beans, and avocado

Dinner: Whole-grain stir-fry with a variety of veggies, tofu, and a homemade sauce

Thursday:

Breakfast: Whole-grain waffles topped with fresh fruit and a drizzle of maple syrup

Lunch: Whole-grain pasta with a homemade tomato sauce, topped with grated Parmesan cheese

Dinner: Whole-grain lasagna with a homemade meat or vegetable sauce

Friday:

Breakfast: Veggie and cheese omelette

Lunch: Whole-grain pizza with a variety of veggies and mozzarella cheese

Dinner: Whole-grain tacos filled with seasoned ground beef or chicken, topped with lettuce, cheese, and salsa

Saturday:

Breakfast: Fresh fruit with a side of yogurt

Lunch: Homemade trail mix with a variety of nuts and dried fruit

Dinner: Grilled fish with a side of quinoa and steamed asparagus

Sunday:

Breakfast: Whole-grain crackers with hummus or avocado spread

Lunch: Whole-grain pita chips with a side of homemade salsa

Dinner: Whole-grain spaghetti with homemade meat or vegetable sauce, topped with grated Parmesan cheese

These are just a few examples of delicious, whole-foods recipes and meal plan.. for more recipes and cook book check

Appendix B

Appendix: Recipes and Meal Plans

Breakfast	Avocado toast with whole grain bread, mashed avocado, and a fried egg	Overnight oats with rolled oats, chia seeds, almond milk, and mixed berries	Veggie scramble with scrambled eggs, bell peppers, onions, and spinach
Lunch	Quinoa and black bean salad with mixed greens, cherry tomatoes, and a lime-cilantro dressing	Whole grain pasta with a homemade marinara sauce, sautéed vegetables, and a sprinkle of Parmesan cheese	Grilled portobello mushrooms topped with a pesto sauce, roasted red pepper, and feta cheese.

Dinner	Lentil and vegetable stew with a mix of carrots, potatoes, and kale in a flavorful tomato broth	Baked salmon with a honey-mustard glaze, served with a quinoa and vegetable medley	Roasted vegetables with a variety of seasonal vegetables, tossed with olive oil and herbs, served with a side of whole-grain bread
Snacks	Apple slices with almond butter	Greek yogurt with honey and berries	Roasted chickpeas

MEAL PLAN TABLE

	Breakfast	Lunch	Dinner	Snack
Monday	Avocado toast	Quinoa and black bean salad	Lentil and vegetable stew	Greek yogurt
Tuesday	Overnight oats	Whole grain pasta	Baked salmon	Roasted chickpeas
Wednesday	Veggie scramble	Grilled portobello mushrooms	Roasted vegetables	Apple slices with almond butter
Thursday	Repeat Monday's meals			
Friday	Repeat Tuesday's meals			
Saturday	Repeat Wednesday's meals			
Sunday	Repeat Monday's meals			

Note: Feel free to mix and match these recipes, and customize them to your liking. Also, make sure to incorporate a variety of fruits and vegetables in your diet, and to drink plenty of water.